Dr Patrick Wisedoc

Master Your Vagus Nerve:

Natural Ability Guide to Heal Anxiety, Depression, Stress, and Trauma Through Nervous System Regulation: Exercises, Techniques, and Practices

Proverbs

"An ounce of prevention is worth a pound of cure."

"A calm sea never made a skilled sailor."

"A healthy mind in a healthy body"

"The journey of a thousand miles begins with a single step."

"Where the mind goes, the energy flows."

Master Your Vagus Nerve:

This book can be your guide! It unlocks the secrets of the vagus nerve, a powerful nerve that acts as a direct line between your brain and your body. By understanding and activating your vagus nerve, you can:

- Reduce stress and anxiety: Learn how to switch off your fight-or-flight response and promote relaxation.
- Improve digestion and gut health: Discover how the vagus nerve influences your digestive system and how to support its proper function.
- Boost your mood and emotional well-being: Explore the link between the vagus nerve and your emotions, and learn techniques to regulate them.
- Enhance sleep quality: Discover how to activate your vagus nerve for deeper, more restful sleep.
- Support overall health and well-being: This book goes beyond stress relief, providing tools to cultivate a calmer, healthier you.

This is your practical guide to understanding your nervous system and unlocking the power within. Take charge of your well-being, one activated vagus nerve at a time!

Master Your Vagus Nerve: Contents

Master Your Vagus Nerve:
Contents

Master Your Vagus Nerve:
Contents

Subsection 1.1: How the Autonomic Nervous System Works

The autonomic nervous system (ANS) is a complex network of nerves that regulates various involuntary bodily functions, like heartbeat, breathing, digestion, and even sweating. It works tirelessly in the background, maintaining a healthy internal environment (homeostasis) without requiring conscious effort. Here's a breakdown of how it functions:

Two Branches, One Goal:

The ANS consists of two main branches with opposing effects:

- **Sympathetic nervous system (fight-or-flight):** This branch activates during stressful situations or emergencies. It increases heart rate, breathing rate, blood pressure, and blood sugar to prepare your body for action.
- **Parasympathetic nervous system (rest-and-digest):** This branch promotes relaxation and supports bodily functions during calmer periods. It slows heart rate, breathing rate, and blood pressure, and aids in digestion and elimination.

Subsection 1.1: How the Autonomic Nervous System Works

Communication Highway:

The ANS uses a complex network of nerves to communicate between the brain and various organs. Here's the general flow of information:

- **Sensory input:** Information about your internal and external environment is gathered by sensory receptors throughout your body.
- **Relay to brainstem:** This sensory information is transmitted to the brainstem, a part of the brain responsible for regulating vital functions.
- **Branch activation:** The brainstem interprets the information and sends signals through the sympathetic or parasympathetic nervous system branches depending on the situation.
- **Organ response:** Organs receive signals from the ANS and adjust their activity accordingly.

Maintaining Balance:

The sympathetic and parasympathetic nervous systems work in a dynamic balance. In a healthy state, they constantly adapt to maintain optimal internal conditions. For instance, during exercise, the sympathetic nervous system might increase your heart rate to deliver more oxygen to your muscles, while the parasympathetic nervous system might work to maintain digestion.

Subsection 1.1: How the Autonomic Nervous System Works

Factors Affecting the ANS:

Several factors can influence the activity of the ANS, including:

- **Stress**: Chronic stress can disrupt the balance between the sympathetic and parasympathetic nervous systems, leading to health problems.
- **Diet**: A balanced diet rich in nutrients can support the overall health of the nervous system.
- **Sleep**: Adequate sleep allows the body to rest and repair, promoting a healthy nervous system.
- **Exercise**: Regular physical activity can help improve the body's response to stress and promote relaxation.

Understanding the ANS can be helpful in managing your overall health and well-being. By incorporating stress-reduction techniques, maintaining a healthy lifestyle, and being mindful of the mind-body connection, you can support the proper functioning of your autonomic nervous system.

Subsection 1.2: The Sympathetic Nervous System (Fight-or-Flight Response)

The sympathetic nervous system (SNS), also known as the fight-or-flight response, is one of the two branches of the autonomic nervous system (ANS) responsible for controlling involuntary bodily functions. Unlike the parasympathetic nervous system (rest-and-digest), the SNS is activated in response to perceived threats or stressful situations, preparing your body for action. Here's a deeper dive into the SNS and its role:

Gearing Up for Action:

Imagine encountering a dangerous situation. The SNS kicks in, triggering a cascade of physiological changes to optimize your body's ability to handle the threat. Here are some key actions it initiates:

- **Increased Heart Rate and Blood Pressure:** The SNS stimulates the heart to pump faster, delivering more oxygen and nutrients to your muscles for action. It also constricts blood vessels, raising blood pressure to prioritize blood flow to vital organs like the brain and muscles.
- **Energy Mobilization:** The SNS triggers the release of hormones like adrenaline (epinephrine) and cortisol. These hormones increase blood sugar levels for readily available energy and break down stored fat for sustained energy.

Subsection 1.2: The Sympathetic Nervous System (Fight-or-Flight Response)

- **Heightened Senses:** The SNS dilates your pupils, sharpening your vision. It also increases your hearing acuity and may make you more aware of your surroundings.
- **Non-essential Functions on Hold:** Digestion, urination, and other non-critical bodily functions are temporarily suppressed to focus resources on immediate survival.
- **Sweat Production:** The SNS stimulates sweat glands to cool your body down during exertion.

Fight, Flight, or Freeze:

While the terms "fight-or-flight" are often used interchangeably with the SNS, recent research suggests a more nuanced response. The SNS can trigger a broader range of reactions depending on the perceived threat and individual differences:

- **Fight:** When facing a direct threat, the SNS prepares your body to physically confront the danger.
- **Flight:** When escape is the best option, the SNS prioritizes mobility and endurance to flee the situation.

Subsection 1.2: The Sympathetic Nervous System (Fight-or-Flight Response)

- **Freeze**: In some cases, the SNS might trigger a freeze response, where you become motionless and appear non-threatening in the hope of avoiding confrontation.

The Importance of Balance:

The SNS plays a vital role in keeping us safe and adaptable. However, chronic stress and constant activation of the SNS can lead to health problems like anxiety, high blood pressure, and digestive issues.

Promoting Balance:

Techniques like deep breathing, meditation, and yoga can help activate the parasympathetic nervous system, promoting relaxation and counteracting the effects of chronic stress. Maintaining a healthy lifestyle with regular exercise, a balanced diet, and adequate sleep also contributes to a well-regulated nervous system.

Understanding the SNS and its role in the fight-or-flight response can empower you to manage stress more effectively and support your overall health and well-being.

Subsection 1.3: The Parasympathetic Nervous System (Rest-and-Digest Response)

The parasympathetic nervous system (PNS), often referred to as the "rest-and-digest" system, is the other half of the autonomic nervous system (ANS) working in beautiful opposition to the sympathetic nervous system (SNS). Unlike the SNS, which gears you up for action, the PNS promotes relaxation, restoration, and essential bodily functions during calmer periods.

Hitting the Brakes:

Imagine yourself in a safe and relaxed environment. The PNS takes center stage, initiating a series of physiological changes to promote well-being:

- **Decreased Heart Rate and Blood Pressure**: The PNS slows your heart rate and relaxes blood vessels, lowering blood pressure. This conserves energy and promotes a sense of calm.
- **Rest and Digest:** The PNS stimulates digestion by increasing saliva production, enhancing gut motility, and promoting efficient nutrient absorption.
- **Conserving Energy:** The PNS promotes the storage of energy by decreasing blood sugar levels and reducing the breakdown of glycogen (stored sugar) in muscles.

Subsection 1.3: The Parasympathetic Nervous System (Rest-and-Digest Response)

- **Tear Production and Mucus Flow**: The PNS increases tear production to lubricate your eyes and stimulates mucus production to keep your respiratory system moist and healthy.
- **Sexual Arousal and Urogenital Function**: The PNS plays a role in sexual arousal and regulates bladder and bowel function.

Promoting Overall Well-being:

The PNS plays a crucial role in maintaining a healthy internal environment and supporting vital bodily functions. Here are some additional benefits of a well-functioning PNS:

- **Improved Sleep**: PNS activity promotes relaxation and prepares the body for restful sleep.
- **Enhanced Immunity**: The PNS plays a role in regulating the immune system, helping your body fight off infections and illnesses.
- **Faster Healing**: Increased blood flow and improved circulation facilitated by the PNS can contribute to faster healing after injuries.

Subsection 1.3: The Parasympathetic Nervous System (Rest-and-Digest Response)

The Importance of Balance:

Just like the SNS, the PNS needs to be in balance with the fight-or-flight response for optimal health. Constant stress and chronic activation of the SNS can disrupt this balance, hindering the PNS from performing its essential functions.

Activating the Relaxation Response:

Techniques like deep breathing exercises, meditation, progressive muscle relaxation, and spending time in nature can all help activate the PNS and promote feelings of calm and well-being.

Understanding the PNS and its role in the rest-and-digest response can empower you to prioritize relaxation techniques and create a lifestyle that supports a healthy nervous system balance.

Subsection 2.1: What is the Vagus Nerve?

The vagus nerve, also known as the tenth cranial nerve (CN X), is the longest and most complex nerve in the autonomic nervous system (ANS). It's like a superhighway carrying information between your brain and various organs throughout your body, playing a critical role in many vital functions. Here's a closer look at this fascinating nerve:

The vagus nerve has a wide range of responsibilities, influencing various bodily functions:

- Digestion: It controls the muscles involved in swallowing, helps regulate stomach acid production, and stimulates gut motility for efficient digestion.
- Heart Rate and Blood Pressure: The vagus nerve can slow down your heart rate and lower blood pressure, promoting relaxation.
- Breathing: It plays a role in regulating breathing rate and depth.
- Inflammation: The vagus nerve has anti-inflammatory properties and helps regulate the body's inflammatory response.
- Voice and Speech: It controls the muscles in your larynx, allowing you to speak and sing.
- Facial Expressions and Taste: The vagus nerve contributes to certain facial expressions and taste perception.

The Vagus Nerve and the Polyvagal Theory:

The polyvagal theory, proposed by Dr. Stephen Porges, expands on our understanding of the vagus nerve. It suggests that the vagus nerve has different branches that support three hierarchically organized states in the nervous system:

- **Social Engagement:** This state is activated when you feel safe and connected. The vagus nerve promotes calmness and allows for social interaction and digestion.
- **Fight-or-Flight:** When faced with a perceived threat, the sympathetic nervous system takes over, and the vagus nerve helps mobilize resources for action.
- **Freeze or Shut Down:** In extreme danger, the vagus nerve might trigger a freeze response, where you become motionless and conserve energy.

The Vagus Nerve and Your Wellbeing:

A healthy vagus nerve tone is associated with several benefits:

- Reduced anxiety and stress
- Improved digestion and gut health
- Stronger immune system
- Better sleep
- Enhanced emotional regulation
- Conversely, a dysregulated vagus nerve might contribute to digestive issues, anxiety, and difficulty relaxing.

Understanding the vagus nerve and its diverse functions can empower you to explore ways to stimulate and support its healthy activity for improved overall well-being.

Subsection 2.2: The Location of the Vagus Nerve

The vagus nerve, also known as the tenth cranial nerve (CN X), is the longest and most complex nerve in the autonomic nervous system (ANS). It originates in the brainstem and travels down both sides of the neck and chest, branching out to innervate (provide nerve supply to) many organs throughout the body. Here's a look at its location:

A Long and Winding Path:

The vagus nerve has a complex pathway, innervating numerous organs and tissues. Here's a simplified overview of its course:

- It emerges from the brainstem and travels down through the jugular foramen, a small opening at the base of the skull.
- It passes through the neck alongside the carotid artery and jugular vein.
- In the chest, it branches out to innervate organs like the heart, lungs, stomach, intestines, and liver.

Bilateral Representation:

The vagus nerve exists on both the left and right sides of the body, with each side innervating the corresponding organs. This bilateral representation ensures redundancy and continued function even if one side is compromised.

Subsection 2.3: The Unique Nervous System – The Polyvagal Theory

The Polyvagal Theory, developed by Dr. Stephen Porges, offers a unique perspective on the autonomic nervous system (ANS), particularly focusing on the role of the vagus nerve. It builds upon our understanding of the fight-or-flight response by suggesting a more nuanced view of how our nervous system responds to threats and promotes social connection.

Here's a breakdown of the Polyvagal Theory:

Hierarchical Response System:

The theory proposes that the ANS has a hierarchical organization, with three progressively complex circuits:

1. **Myelinated Ventral Vagal Complex (Social Engagement System):** This is the newest circuit evolutionarily. It involves the myelinated portion of the vagus nerve and is responsible for our social engagement response. When activated, it promotes feelings of safety, connection, and well-being. This circuit allows the vagus nerve to slow heart rate, promote digestion, and support vocal communication.

Subsection 2.3: The Unique Nervous System – The Polyvagal Theory

2. Sympathetic Nervous System (Fight-or-Flight System): This familiar system is activated in response to perceived threats. It prepares the body for action by increasing heart rate, blood pressure, and energy mobilization.

3. Dorsal Vagal Complex (Freeze or Shut Down System): This is the most primitive circuit and is activated in situations of extreme danger when escape or fight seem impossible. The vagus nerve, in this state, might trigger a freeze response where the body becomes motionless, conserving energy and appearing non-threatening. In extreme cases, it can even lead to fainting.

Evolutionary Advantage:

The Polyvagal Theory suggests that these circuits evolved sequentially, with the social engagement system being the most recent development. This layered structure allows for a flexible response system. We can first attempt social cues (communication) to resolve a threat, then mobilize for fight-or-flight if needed, and finally resort to a freeze response as a last resort.

Subsection 2.3: The Unique Nervous System – The Polyvagal Theory

Implications for Wellbeing:

Understanding the Polyvagal Theory can be helpful for managing stress and anxiety. By actively engaging the social engagement system through practices like mindfulness, meditation, and connecting with others, we can promote feelings of safety and well-being. Techniques like deep breathing and stimulating the vagus nerve (discussed later in the book) can also contribute to a sense of calm and reduce the dominance of the fight-or-flight response.

The Polyvagal Theory provides a fascinating lens through which to understand our nervous system's response to the environment. By recognizing these different circuits and their functions, we can take a more proactive approach to managing stress and promoting overall well-being.

Subsection 2.3: The Unique Nervous System – The Polyvagal Theory

The Polyvagal Theory Framework

The Polyvagal Theory, proposed by Dr. Stephen Porges, offers a unique perspective on the autonomic nervous system (ANS), particularly focusing on the role of the vagus nerve. It builds upon the fight-or-flight response by suggesting a more nuanced view of how our nervous system prioritizes safety, social connection, and survival.

Key Concepts:

Hierarchical Organization:
The ANS is organized in a hierarchy, with three progressively complex circuits:

- 1. Myelinated Ventral Vagal Complex (Social Engagement System): This is the newest circuit evolutionarily. It promotes feelings of safety, connection, and well-being. This system allows us to slow heart rate, promote digestion, and support vocal communication.
- 2. Sympathetic Nervous System (Fight-or-Flight System): This familiar system prepares the body for action in response to perceived threats.

Subsection 2.3: The Unique Nervous System – The Polyvagal Theory

3. Dorsal Vagal Complex (Freeze or Shut Down System): This is the most primitive circuit, activated in extreme danger when escape or fight seem impossible. It triggers a freeze response for conservation or fainting as a last resort.

Vagus Nerve Involvement:

The vagus nerve plays a central role in two circuits:
* Social Engagement System: The myelinated ventral vagus nerve branch promotes feelings of safety and connection.
* Dorsal Vagal Complex: In extreme situations, the vagus nerve might trigger a freeze response.

Evolutionary Advantage:

The theory suggests these circuits evolved sequentially, with the social engagement system being the most recent development. This layered structure allows for a flexible response system, attempting social cues first, then fight-or-flight, and finally freeze as a last resort.

Subsection 2.3: The Unique Nervous System – The Polyvagal Theory

Benefits of Understanding the Polyvagal Theory:

- **Stress Management**: By recognizing the different circuits and their functions, we can identify triggers and choose appropriate responses.
- **Mindfulness and Meditation:** The theory highlights the importance of the social engagement system, which mindfulness and meditation practices can activate to promote feelings of safety and well-being.
- **Social Connection:** Understanding the vagus nerve's role in social engagement underscores the importance of positive social interactions for overall well-being.

The Polyvagal Theory is a valuable framework for understanding the connection between our nervous system, environment, and mental and physical health. By incorporating practices that activate the social engagement system and promote vagus nerve activity, we can cultivate resilience and well-being.

The Functions of the Vagus Nerve (Physiology)

The vagus nerve, also known as the tenth cranial nerve (CN X), is the longest and most complex nerve in the autonomic nervous system (ANS). It acts like a superhighway carrying messages between your brain and various organs throughout your body, influencing a wide range of physiological functions. Here's a closer look at the vagus nerve's key roles:

Digestive Maestro:

- **Swallowing**: The vagus nerve controls the muscles involved in swallowing, ensuring smooth passage of food from the mouth to the stomach.
- **Stomach Acid Production**: It helps regulate stomach acid production, important for digestion but needing control to prevent ulcers.
- **Gut Motility**: The vagus nerve stimulates the muscles in your intestines, promoting efficient movement of food for proper digestion and nutrient absorption.

Heart and Circulation:

Heart Rate and Blood Pressure: The vagus nerve plays a crucial role in slowing down your heart rate and lowering blood pressure, promoting relaxation and counteracting the effects of the fight-or-flight response.

Respiratory Regulator:

- **Breathing Rate and Depth:** The vagus nerve influences the rate and depth of your breathing. It helps regulate a calm and steady breathing pattern.

Anti-inflammatory Champion:

- **Inflammation Modulation:** The vagus nerve has anti-inflammatory properties. It can dampen excessive inflammatory responses throughout the body, contributing to overall health.

Vocal Cords and Speech:

- **Laryngeal Muscle Control:** The vagus nerve controls the muscles in your larynx, allowing you to speak and sing by adjusting the tension of your vocal cords.

Beyond the Basics:

The vagus nerve's influence extends beyond these core functions. It also plays a role in:

- Facial Expressions and Taste: The vagus nerve contributes to certain facial expressions and taste perception.
- Ear Function: It might influence some aspects of hearing and earwax production.
- Insulin Regulation: The vagus nerve may be involved in insulin signaling and blood sugar control.
- The vagus nerve's versatility makes it a critical player in maintaining a healthy internal environment (homeostasis).

Chapter 4: The Impact of the Nervous System on Your Emotions

The nervous system plays a fundamental role in shaping our emotions. It acts as a complex communication network, constantly sending and receiving signals between the brain and the body. Here's how the nervous system influences our emotional experience:

The Autonomic Nervous System (ANS) Takes Center Stage:

The ANS, a major division of the nervous system, is particularly influential in emotions. It has two branches that work in opposition:

- **Sympathetic** Nervous System (Fight-or-Flight): When faced with a perceived threat or stressful situation, the sympathetic nervous system kicks in. It triggers physiological changes like increased heart rate, breathing rate, and blood pressure, preparing your body for action. These physical changes can manifest as feelings of anxiety, arousal, or even fear.

Chapter 4: The Impact of the Nervous System on Your Emotions

Parasympathetic Nervous System (Rest-and-Digest): In contrast, the parasympathetic nervous system promotes relaxation and a sense of calm. It slows down heart rate, breathing, and blood pressure, allowing the body to conserve energy and focus on digestion and other vital functions. This activation can contribute to feelings of peace, contentment, and safety.

The Limbic System: Processing Center for Emotions:

The limbic system, a group of structures deep within the brain, plays a crucial role in processing emotions. It receives signals from various sensory inputs (sight, sound, touch, etc.) and interprets them based on past experiences and memories. This interpretation triggers emotional responses that are then communicated to the body through the ANS.

Chapter 4: The Impact of the Nervous System on Your Emotions

The Feedback Loop:

The relationship between the nervous system and emotions is a two-way street:

- **Emotions Impact the Nervous System:** Our emotions can directly influence the ANS. For example, feeling anxious can trigger the fight-or-flight response, leading to physical changes like a racing heart.

- **Nervous System Impacts Emotions:** Conversely, the nervous system's activity can influence our emotional state. For instance, a rapid heart rate and shallow breathing, triggered by the fight-or-flight response, can intensify feelings of anxiety.

The Role of Neurotransmitters:

Neurotransmitters are chemical messengers that facilitate communication between brain cells. Different neurotransmitters play specific roles in emotional experiences.

- **Dopamine:** Associated with pleasure and reward.
- **Serotonin:** Contributes to feelings of happiness and well-being.
- **Norepinephrine:** Involved in alertness and arousal, can also contribute to anxiety.
- **GABA:** Promotes relaxation and calmness.

Chapter 4: The Impact of the Nervous System on Your Emotions

The activity of these neurotransmitters, influenced by the nervous system, shapes our emotional responses.

Understanding this intricate interplay between the nervous system and emotions can empower you to manage your emotional well-being. Techniques like mindfulness meditation, deep breathing, and managing stress can help promote activity in the parasympathetic nervous system and contribute to a calmer emotional state.

The vagus nerve, due to its extensive influence throughout the body, can be susceptible to various dysfunctions. These dysfunctions can manifest in a wide range of symptoms depending on the specific area affected. Here's a breakdown of some potential vagus nerve dysfunctions:

Gastrointestinal Issues:

- Gastroparesis: This condition involves delayed stomach emptying due to impaired vagus nerve function. Symptoms include nausea, vomiting, bloating, and abdominal pain.
- Gastroesophageal Reflux Disease (GERD): A weakened lower esophageal sphincter, partially controlled by the vagus nerve, can contribute to GERD, causing heartburn and acid reflux.
- Constipation: Vagus nerve dysfunction can disrupt gut motility, leading to constipation and difficulty passing stool.

Digestive Problems – Additional Considerations:

- Vagus nerve dysfunction might also contribute to issues like irritable bowel syndrome (IBS) and difficulty swallowing (dysphagia).
- These conditions can have overlapping symptoms, and proper diagnosis by a healthcare professional is crucial.

Heart and Circulatory Problems:

- **Postural Orthostatic Tachycardia Syndrome (POTS):** This condition involves dizziness or fainting upon standing due to a drop in blood pressure and may be linked to vagus nerve dysfunction.
- **Arrhythmias**: In some cases, vagus nerve dysfunction might contribute to irregular heart rhythms.

Respiratory Issues:

- Chronic cough: Vagus nerve irritation can sometimes trigger a persistent cough.

Other Potential Manifestations:

- Hoarseness or vocal problems: The vagus nerve controls the muscles in the larynx, and dysfunction can affect vocal quality.
- Digestive bloating and pain: A general discomfort or tightness in the abdomen due to vagus nerve issues.
- Difficulty relaxing: The vagus nerve plays a role in the parasympathetic nervous system's "rest-and-digest" function. Dysfunction can make it challenging to achieve relaxation.

Important Notes:

- Diagnosing vagus nerve dysfunction can be complex because symptoms often overlap with other conditions.
- Consulting a healthcare professional for proper evaluation is essential.
- Vagus nerve dysfunction can sometimes be caused by underlying health conditions like diabetes or autoimmune diseases.
- While these are some potential consequences of vagus nerve dysfunction, it's important to remember that a diagnosis should be made by a qualified medical professional. There may be other explanations for your symptoms.

The vagus nerve, with its widespread influence on the body, can benefit from various approaches to promote its health and potentially alleviate symptoms associated with dysfunction. Here's a look at some methods:

Lifestyle Practices:

- **Stress Management:** Chronic stress can negatively impact the vagus nerve. Techniques like mindfulness meditation, deep breathing exercises, yoga, and spending time in nature can help manage stress and promote vagus nerve activity.

- **Dietary Adjustments:** A balanced diet rich in fruits, vegetables, and whole grains provides essential nutrients to support nervous system health. Limiting processed foods, added sugars, and unhealthy fats may also be beneficial.

- **Regular Exercise:** Physical activity, particularly aerobic exercise, can stimulate the vagus nerve and improve its overall function.

- **Sleep Hygiene:** Prioritizing good sleep allows your body to rest and repair, promoting vagus nerve health. Establishing a regular sleep schedule and creating a relaxing bedtime routine can contribute to better sleep quality.

- **Cold Exposure:** Short-term cold exposure, such as cold showers or ice packs applied briefly to the face and neck, can activate the vagus nerve and promote feelings of alertness and well-being.

Supportive Therapies:

- **Craniosacral Therapy:** This gentle manual therapy focuses on releasing restrictions in the fascia (connective tissue) around the head, neck, and spine, which may indirectly support vagus nerve function.

- **Acupuncture:** Acupuncture may stimulate the vagus nerve through specific needle placements, potentially promoting relaxation and reducing inflammation.

- **Biofeedback:** Biofeedback can help you learn to control certain bodily functions, like heart rate and breathing, which can indirectly influence vagus nerve activity.

Naturopathic Approaches:

Certain supplements, like Vitamin B complex and probiotics, may be helpful in supporting nervous system health, but it's crucial to consult with a healthcare professional before starting any supplements.

Medical Interventions:

In some cases, vagus nerve dysfunction may require medical interventions. This could involve medications or, in rare cases, vagus nerve stimulation (VNS) therapy, which uses electrical impulses to stimulate the nerve. However, these approaches are typically considered after exploring more conservative options.

Important Considerations:

- While these approaches hold promise, research on their effectiveness in treating vagus nerve dysfunction is ongoing.
- Consulting a qualified healthcare professional is essential to determine the best course of action for your specific situation.
- They can help identify any underlying causes of vagus nerve dysfunction and develop a personalized treatment plan.
- Remember, healing vagus nerve dysfunction often involves a multifaceted approach. By incorporating lifestyle changes, exploring supportive therapies, and consulting a healthcare professional, you can take steps to promote vagus nerve health and potentially improve your overall well-being.

The vagus nerve, with its far-reaching influence on our bodies, deserves some TLC. Here's a roadmap to create a daily routine that can support vagus nerve health and potentially enhance your overall well-being:

Morning Rituals to Spark Vagus Nerve Activity:

- **Gentle Movement:** Start your day with gentle stretches, yoga, or a light walk. This activates the nervous system and promotes blood flow, both beneficial for the vagus nerve.
- **Deep Breathing Exercises:** Dedicate 5-10 minutes to deep, diaphragmatic breathing. Inhale slowly through your nose and exhale completely through your mouth. This can activate the parasympathetic nervous system (rest-and-digest) and counter the effects of stress.
- **Cold Exposure (Optional):** If you're brave enough, try a cold shower or splash cold water on your face. This short-term cold exposure can stimulate the vagus nerve and leave you feeling energized.

Nourishing Practices Throughout the Day:

- Mindful Eating: Savor your meals, chew thoroughly, and avoid distractions while eating. This promotes digestion and reduces stress, both of which benefit the vagus nerve.
- Hydration: Drink plenty of water throughout the day. Dehydration can negatively impact the nervous system, so stay hydrated to support optimal vagus nerve function.
- Social Connection: Engage in positive social interactions with loved ones or friends. Social connection activates the social engagement system of the vagus nerve, promoting feelings of safety and well-being.
- Laughter is Medicine: Find humor in your day! Laughter is a powerful tool that can stimulate the vagus nerve and reduce stress hormones.

Winding Down for a Restful Night:

- Dim the Lights: An hour before bedtime, dim the lights in your environment. This helps suppress melatonin production, the sleep hormone, and prepares your body for relaxation.
- Relaxation Techniques: Engage in calming activities like reading, meditation, or light stretching before bed. These practices promote relaxation and signal to your body that it's time to wind down, activating the parasympathetic nervous system.
- Digital Detox: Avoid screen time (phones, laptops) for at least an hour before bed. The blue light emitted from electronic devices can disrupt sleep patterns and negatively impact vagus nerve function.
- Soothing Sounds: Listen to calming music or nature sounds to promote relaxation and prepare your body for sleep.

Bonus Tips:

- Probiotic-Rich Foods: Incorporate yogurt, kimchi, kombucha, and other probiotic-rich foods into your diet. Probiotics may support a healthy gut microbiome, which can indirectly benefit the vagus nerve.
- Singing or Humming: Singing or humming activates the vagus nerve and can be a fun way to promote relaxation.
- Gratitude Practice: Take a few minutes each day to reflect on things you're grateful for. Gratitude practices can promote positive emotions and contribute to vagus nerve health.

Remember: Consistency is key! By incorporating these practices into your daily routine, you can create a foundation for a healthy vagus nerve and potentially experience improved digestion, reduced stress, better sleep, and overall well-being.

It's important to note that these practices are meant to be supportive and not a replacement for professional medical advice. If you suspect vagus nerve dysfunction, consult a healthcare professional for proper diagnosis and a personalized treatment plan.

While directly stimulating the vagus nerve through food choices isn't entirely possible, there are dietary strategies that can indirectly support its function by promoting a healthy gut and reducing inflammation. Here's a look at some "better" food choices for vagus nerve health:

Fiber Powerhouses:

- Fruits and Vegetables: A diet rich in fruits and vegetables provides essential vitamins, minerals, and fiber. Fiber acts as a prebiotic, feeding the good bacteria in your gut which can have positive downstream effects on the vagus nerve.
- Whole Grains: Opt for whole grains like brown rice, quinoa, and oats over refined grains. Whole grains are a good source of fiber and complex carbohydrates, which can promote gut health and overall well-being.

Fermented Friends:

Probiotic-Rich Foods: Include fermented foods like yogurt, kimchi, kombucha, kefir, and sauerkraut in your diet. These foods contain probiotics, live bacteria that contribute to a healthy gut microbiome. A healthy gut microbiome can positively influence the vagus nerve through the gut-brain connection.

Omega-3 Rich Choices:

- **Fatty Fish**: Salmon, mackerel, sardines, and herring are excellent sources of omega-3 fatty acids. Omega-3s have anti-inflammatory properties and may contribute to overall nervous system health, including the vagus nerve.

Hydration Hero:

- **Water**: Staying hydrated is crucial for optimal bodily function, including nervous system health. Aim to drink plenty of water throughout the day to support vagus nerve function.

Foods to Limit:

- Processed Foods: Processed foods are often high in unhealthy fats, added sugars, and refined carbohydrates. These can contribute to inflammation and potentially disrupt gut health, both of which can negatively impact the vagus nerve.
- Added Sugars: Excessive sugar intake can disrupt gut health and contribute to inflammation. Limiting sugary drinks, sweets, and processed foods is beneficial.

- **Excessive Alcohol:** While moderate alcohol consumption might not be detrimental, heavy alcohol intake can negatively impact the nervous system, including the vagus nerve.

Additional Considerations:

- Individual Needs: Consider any dietary restrictions or allergies you may have when incorporating these suggestions.
- Consult a Nutritionist: A registered dietitian or nutritionist can help create a personalized plan that caters to your specific needs and preferences.

Remember: A balanced and varied diet rich in fruits, vegetables, whole grains, and healthy fats is essential for overall health, which can indirectly support vagus nerve function. By incorporating these suggestions and limiting inflammatory foods, you can create a dietary foundation that promotes a healthy gut and potentially improves vagus nerve health.

Subsection 8.1: The Link Between Human Emotions and Vagus Nerve Functioning

The vagus nerve plays a crucial role in the two-way street between our emotions and our bodies. Here's a breakdown of this fascinating connection:

The Vagus Nerve: A Key Player in the Emotional Highway:

- **The Parasympathetic Nervous System Conductor:** The vagus nerve is a major component of the parasympathetic nervous system, often referred to as the "rest-and-digest" system. When activated, the vagus nerve promotes feelings of calm, safety, and well-being.

- **The Gut-Brain Connection:** The vagus nerve directly connects the gut and the brain. A healthy gut microbiome, influenced by diet and lifestyle factors, can send signals to the brain via the vagus nerve, promoting feelings of calmness and contentment. Conversely, an unhealthy gut microbiome can send signals that contribute to anxiety and stress.

Subsection 8.1: The Link Between Human Emotions and Vagus Nerve Functioning

How Emotions Influence the Vagus Nerve:

- **Stress and Anxiety:** Chronic stress and anxiety can lead to a dominance of the sympathetic nervous system (fight-or-flight) and suppress the parasympathetic nervous system. This can weaken vagus nerve activity, potentially contributing to digestive issues, difficulty relaxing, and even heartburn.

- **Positive Emotions:** Positive emotions like happiness, gratitude, and social connection can activate the parasympathetic nervous system and strengthen vagus nerve function. This can lead to feelings of calm, improved digestion, and overall well-being.

The Feedback Loop:

The relationship between emotions and the vagus nerve is a continuous cycle:

- **Emotions Impact Vagus Nerve:** Our emotions can directly influence the vagus nerve's activity. For example, feeling stressed can suppress vagus nerve function and lead to physical consequences.

- **Vagus Nerve Impacts Emotions:** The vagus nerve's activity also influences our emotions. For instance, a slow heart rate and relaxed breathing, mediated by the vagus nerve, can promote feelings of calm.

The Impact on Mental Health:

A healthy vagus nerve is crucial for emotional regulation. When the vagus nerve is functioning optimally, it can help us cope with stress, recover from emotional challenges, and experience positive emotions more fully. Conversely, dysfunction in the vagus nerve may be linked to conditions like anxiety and depression.

Enhancing the Vagus Nerve for Emotional Well-being:

By incorporating practices that support vagus nerve health, we can potentially improve our emotional well-being:

- **Stress Management Techniques:** Mindfulness meditation, deep breathing exercises, and spending time in nature can help manage stress and promote vagus nerve activity.
- **Healthy Diet:** A balanced diet rich in fruits, vegetables, whole grains, and healthy fats can contribute to a healthy gut microbiome, indirectly supporting vagus nerve function and potentially influencing emotions.
- **Social Connection:** Prioritizing positive social interactions can activate the vagus nerve's social engagement system and promote feelings of safety and well-being.

Remember, the vagus nerve plays a significant role in the complex dance between our emotions and our physical state. By understanding this connection and taking steps to support vagus nerve health, we can cultivate emotional resilience and promote overall well-being.

Subsection 8.2: How to Control Your Emotions Using the Vagus Nerve

While the vagus nerve plays a significant role in our emotional state, it's important to understand that it's not a direct control panel for emotions. However, by supporting vagus nerve health, you can create a foundation for better emotional regulation. Here's how:

Indirect Influence:

The vagus nerve's influence on emotions is indirect but significant. It's part of the parasympathetic nervous system, which promotes feelings of calm and well-being. Here's how it works:

- **Reduced Stress Response:** When the vagus nerve is active, it helps counter the "fight-or-flight" response triggered by the sympathetic nervous system. This can lead to a decrease in heart rate, blood pressure, and feelings of anxiety.

- **Improved Gut-Brain Connection:** The vagus nerve directly connects the gut and the brain. A healthy gut microbiome, influenced by diet and lifestyle, can send signals to the brain via the vagus nerve, promoting feelings of calmness and contentment.

Strategies to Support Vagus Nerve Health:

By incorporating these practices, you can potentially create a more favorable environment for vagus nerve function, which may indirectly contribute to better emotional regulation:

- **Deep Breathing Exercises:** Deep, diaphragmatic breathing activates the parasympathetic nervous system and can help calm the body and mind.
- **Mindfulness Meditation:** Mindfulness practices can help manage stress and promote emotional awareness, which can be beneficial for emotional regulation.
- **Relaxation Techniques:** Activities like yoga, progressive muscle relaxation, and spending time in nature can promote relaxation and support vagus nerve function.
- **Healthy Diet:** A balanced diet rich in fruits, vegetables, whole grains, and healthy fats can contribute to a healthy gut microbiome, indirectly supporting vagus nerve health and potentially influencing emotions.
- **Social Connection:** Prioritizing positive social interactions can activate the vagus nerve's social engagement system and promote feelings of safety and well-being.

Important Considerations:

- **Consistency is Key:** The benefits of these practices often accumulate over time. Consistent practice is crucial for optimal results.
- **Seeking Professional Help:** For managing strong emotions or mental health concerns, consulting a therapist or counselor is highly recommended. They can provide personalized strategies for emotional regulation.

The vagus nerve is a powerful player in our overall well-being, but it's not a magic bullet for emotional control. However, by taking steps to support its health, you can create a foundation for better emotional regulation and experience a calmer, more balanced emotional state.

Vagus nerve stimulation (VNS) has emerged as a promising therapeutic approach for treating various neurological and mental health conditions. Here's a breakdown of its potential benefits:

Applications of VNS:

VNS involves implanting a small device near the left vagus nerve in the chest. The device delivers electrical pulses to the nerve, influencing its activity. While the exact mechanisms are still being explored, VNS offers potential benefits for several conditions:

- **Epilepsy**: VNS therapy has been approved by the FDA as a treatment for epilepsy that is difficult to control with medications. It can help reduce the frequency and severity of seizures.

- **Depression**: Research suggests VNS may be a helpful treatment option for people with treatment-resistant depression, particularly those who haven't responded well to traditional medications.

- **Other Conditions:** VNS is being investigated for its potential role in treating other conditions like chronic pain, migraines, and even tinnitus (ringing in the ears).

How VNS May Work:

The precise way VNS exerts its effects is still under investigation, but some potential mechanisms include:

- **Modulating Brain Activity:** VNS may influence the electrical activity in the brain, particularly areas involved in mood regulation and seizure control.

- **Anti-inflammatory Effects:** VNS might have anti-inflammatory properties that could benefit conditions like epilepsy and depression.

- **Neuromodulation:** VNS may help regulate the nervous system's overall activity, promoting a balance between the sympathetic and parasympathetic systems.

Benefits of VNS Therapy:

- **Minimally Invasive:** Compared to traditional brain surgeries, VNS is a minimally invasive procedure with a shorter recovery time.

- **Adjustable Settings:** The VNS device can be programmed to deliver electrical pulses at specific frequencies and intensities, allowing for customization based on individual needs.

- **Long-Term Potential:** VNS therapy can offer long-term benefits for some conditions, with effects potentially improving over time.

- **Relatively Safe:** VNS is generally well-tolerated, with side effects like hoarseness or voice changes typically mild and manageable.

Important Considerations:

- **Not a Cure:** VNS is not a cure for any condition, but rather a therapeutic tool that can help manage symptoms.

Subsection 8.3: The Benefits of Vagus Nerve Stimulation

- **Individualized Treatment:** VNS is not suitable for everyone. Consulting with a healthcare professional is crucial to determine if VNS is a viable treatment option.

- **Long-Term Commitment:** VNS therapy often requires a long-term commitment, as the device remains implanted.

- **Ongoing Research:** Research on VNS and its applications is ongoing. While promising, more studies are needed to fully understand its long-term effects for various conditions.

Overall, vagus nerve stimulation offers a valuable tool for managing certain neurological and mental health conditions. If you're struggling with a condition that might benefit from VNS, speak with your doctor to discuss the potential risks and benefits and see if this approach is right for you.

Somatic meditation is a mindfulness practice that focuses on bodily sensations and internal experiences rather than thoughts or emotions. It aims to cultivate a deeper sense of connection with your physical being and improve your body awareness.

Here's a breakdown of somatic meditation:

- **Focus on the Body:** Unlike traditional meditation that focuses on quieting the mind, somatic meditation encourages you to pay attention to your physical sensations. This might include noticing tightness in your muscles, the feeling of your breath moving through your body, or even subtle temperature changes in your skin.

- **Body Scan:** A common somatic meditation technique involves a systematic body scan. You mentally scan your body from head to toe, focusing on the sensations in each body part without judgment.

- **Emotions and Sensations:** Somatic meditation acknowledges the connection between physical sensations and emotions. By tuning into your body, you might become aware of underlying emotional states you weren't consciously experiencing.

- Acceptance and Non-Judgment: A core principle of somatic meditation is acceptance and non-judgment. You observe your bodily sensations without trying to change them or judge them as good or bad.

Benefits of Somatic Meditation:

- Reduced Stress and Anxiety: By focusing on the present moment and your body, somatic meditation can help reduce stress and anxiety.

- Improved Body Awareness: This practice can lead to a deeper understanding of your body's signals, allowing you to better manage pain and discomfort.

- Emotional Regulation: By connecting with your physical sensations, you can become more aware of your emotions and develop healthier coping mechanisms.

- Enhanced Self-Compassion: Somatic meditation fosters self-compassion by encouraging acceptance of your bodily experiences.

Getting Started with Somatic Meditation:

Here are some tips for trying somatic meditation:

- **Find a Quiet Place:** Choose a quiet and comfortable place where you won't be interrupted.

- **Comfortable Position:** Sit or lie down in a comfortable position that allows you to relax.

- **Close Your Eyes (Optional):** You can close your eyes to focus inward, but keeping them open can also be helpful for some.

- **Body Scan:** Begin by focusing on your breath. Then, slowly scan your body from head to toe, noticing any sensations you experience.

- **Non-Judgmental Observation:** Observe your sensations without judgment. If your mind wanders, gently bring your attention back to your body.

- **Start Small:** Begin with short practice sessions (5–10 minutes) and gradually increase the duration as you become more comfortable.

Additional Resources:

There are many guided somatic meditations available online and in apps. You can also find somatic meditation workshops or classes led by experienced practitioners.

Remember, somatic meditation is a practice, and like any skill, it takes time and effort to develop. Be patient with yourself and focus on the experience rather than achieving a specific outcome. By incorporating somatic meditation into your routine, you can cultivate a deeper connection with your body and experience a greater sense of well-being.

Foundational breathing techniques are the cornerstones of breathwork practices. They focus on establishing a slow, deep, and controlled breathing pattern that activates the parasympathetic nervous system (rest-and-digest system) and promotes relaxation. Here are three key techniques to get you started:

1. Diaphragmatic Breathing (Belly Breathing):

This is the most fundamental breathing technique and the foundation for many others. Here's how to do it:

- Find a Comfortable Position: Sit or lie down in a comfortable position with your spine relatively straight. You can place one hand on your belly and the other on your chest.
- Focus on the Breath: Close your eyes gently if that feels comfortable. Begin to focus on your breath.
- Inhale Slowly Through Your Nose: As you inhale, feel your belly expand, pushing your hand outwards. Aim for a slow and deep inhalation, filling your lower lungs with air.
- Relaxed Exhalation Through Nose or Mouth: Purse your lips slightly if exhaling through your mouth. Feel your belly sink inwards as you exhale slowly and completely.

Subsection 9.2: Foundational Breathing Techniques

- Focus on the Cycle: Pay attention to the natural rise and fall of your abdomen as you breathe.
- Practice: Start with short sessions (5–10 minutes) and gradually increase the duration as you become comfortable.

2. Alternate Nostril Breathing (Nadi Shodhana):

This technique involves breathing through one nostril at a time and is believed to balance the hemispheres of the brain. Here's how to do it:

- Find a Comfortable Seated Position: Sit comfortably with your spine straight.
- Close Your Right Nostril: Use your thumb to gently close your right nostril.
- Inhale Slowly Through Left Nostril: Inhale slowly and deeply through your left nostril.
- Hold (Optional): You can hold your breath for a brief moment at the peak of your inhalation (hold comfortably, not forcefully).
- Close Left Nostril and Exhale Through Right: Close your left nostril with your ring finger and exhale slowly through your right nostril.
- Inhale Through Right Nostril: Inhale slowly through your right nostril.

- **Hold (Optional):** Hold your breath for a brief moment at the peak of your inhalation.
- **Exhale Through Left Nostril:** Close your right nostril with your thumb and exhale slowly through your left nostril.
- **Repeat:** Continue alternating inhalations and exhalations through each nostril for several cycles.

3. 4-7-8 Breathing:

This technique combines breath control with visualization and is known for its calming effect. Here's how to do it:

- **Find a Comfortable Seated Position:** Sit comfortably with your spine straight.
- **Prepare to Exhale:** Purse your lips slightly and exhale completely through your mouth, making a whooshing sound.
- **Silent Inhale Through Nose:** Close your mouth and inhale silently through your nose for a count of four.
- **Hold Your Breath:** Hold your breath for a count of seven.
- **Exhale Through Mouth:** Purse your lips again and exhale completely through your mouth for a count of eight, making a whooshing sound.
- **Repeat:** Continue this cycle of inhaling for four, holding for seven, and exhaling for eight for several cycles.

Benefits of Foundational Breathing Techniques:

- Reduced Stress and Anxiety: By activating the parasympathetic nervous system, these techniques can promote relaxation and reduce stress and anxiety.
- Improved Sleep Quality: Slow, deep breaths can signal to the body that it's time to wind down, promoting better sleep.
- Enhanced Focus and Concentration: Focused breathing can improve concentration and mental clarity.
- Lower Blood Pressure: Regular breathwork practice may contribute to lower blood pressure.

Remember: Consistency is key! Regularly practicing these techniques can help you reap their benefits and develop a healthy breathing habit that supports your overall well-being.

Subsection 9.3: Improving Flexibility and Mobility Exercises (pelvic tilts, spinal twists, gentle backbends, butterfly pose, cross-lateral movements)

Here's a sample routine incorporating the exercises you mentioned to improve your flexibility and mobility:

Warm-up (5-10 minutes):

- Light Cardio: Begin with 5-10 minutes of light cardio like brisk walking, jumping jacks, or jogging on the spot. This helps elevate your heart rate and prepare your muscles for movement.
- Dynamic Stretches: Perform dynamic stretches like arm circles, leg swings, and torso twists to gently increase your range of motion.

Mobility Exercises (10-15 minutes per side):

1. Pelvic Tilts:

- Lie on your back with knees bent and feet flat on the floor.
- Engage your core by gently pressing your lower back into the ground.
- Tilt your pelvis anteriorly (arching your lower back) and posteriorly (flattening your lower back) a few times, focusing on the movement in your hips.
- Keep your core engaged throughout the exercise.

*Subsection 9.3: Improving Flexibility and Mobility Exercises
(pelvic tilts, spinal twists, gentle backbends, butterfly pose,
cross-lateral movements)*

2. Spinal Twists:

- Sit on the floor with knees bent and feet flat.
- Extend your right arm out straight with your palm on the floor behind you.
- Twist your torso to the left, looking over your left shoulder. Keep your hips facing forward and avoid arching your back.
- Hold for a breath or two, then repeat on the other side.

3. Gentle Backbends:

- Kneel on the floor with your toes together and knees hip-width apart.
- Sit back on your heels and lean your torso forward, reaching your arms overhead.
- Gently arch your back and feel the stretch in your chest and shoulders. Hold for a breath or two.
- Avoid straining and come back up slowly when you're finished.
- Flexibility Exercises (15–20 minutes per side):

Subsection 9.3: Improving Flexibility and Mobility Exercises (pelvic tilts, spinal twists, gentle backbends, butterfly pose, cross-lateral movements)

4. Butterfly Pose:

- Sit on the floor with the soles of your feet together and knees bent out to the sides.
- Gently press your knees down towards the floor, keeping your back straight.
- Hold for 30 seconds to 1 minute, focusing on the stretch in your inner thighs and groin.

5. Cross-Lateral Movements:

- Stand tall with your feet hip-width apart.
- Reach your right arm overhead and bend sideways to the left, reaching your left hand towards your shin or ankle (avoid rounding your back).
- Hold for 30 seconds to 1 minute, then repeat on the other side.

Cool-down (5-10 minutes):

- Static Stretches: Hold static stretches for each major muscle group you worked on for 30-60 seconds. Focus on deep breathing throughout the stretches.

Subsection 9.3: Improving Flexibility and Mobility Exercises (pelvic tilts, spinal twists, gentle backbends, butterfly pose, cross-lateral movements)

Progression:

As you gain flexibility, you can hold the stretches for longer or increase the number of repetitions.
You can also explore more challenging variations of these exercises.

Important Considerations:

- Listen to your body: Don't push yourself to the point of pain. Stop if you feel any sharp pains and adjust the intensity of the exercises accordingly.
- Breathe: Breathe deeply and steadily throughout the exercises.
- Maintain good form: Focus on proper form to avoid injuries.

Remember: Consistency is key! Regularly performing these exercises will help you improve your flexibility and mobility over time. You may also want to consider consulting a certified personal trainer or physical therapist for a personalized program tailored to your specific needs and goals.

Sound and vibration techniques offer a drug-free approach to pain management and relaxation. Here's a breakdown of two main categories:

1. Sound Therapy:

- **Mechanism**: Sound therapy uses audible sounds to influence the nervous system and promote relaxation or pain relief. Different sounds can have varying effects.

Applications:

- Music Therapy: Listening to calming music can promote relaxation, reduce stress, and potentially manage chronic pain.

- Binaural Beats: These are auditory illusions created by presenting slightly different tones to each ear. Binaural beats can influence brainwave activity and promote relaxation, focus, or sleep.

- Nature Sounds: Listening to calming nature sounds like waves crashing or birds chirping can reduce stress and promote relaxation.

2. Vibration Therapy:

Mechanism: Vibration therapy applies mechanical vibrations to the body, targeting specific areas or delivered whole-body. It's thought to work by:

- Gate Control Theory: Vibrations may stimulate nerve fibers, "gating out" pain signals from reaching the brain.
- Increased Blood Flow: Vibration can improve blood circulation, potentially aiding in muscle recovery and reducing pain.
- Reduced Muscle Spasticity: Vibration therapy may help relax tense muscles, reducing stiffness and discomfort.

Applications:

- Massage Therapy: Massage therapists often use vibration tools to target muscle tension and promote relaxation.

- Percussive Therapy: Handheld percussion devices deliver rapid pulses to target muscle soreness and tightness.

- Whole Body Vibration (WBV): Standing on a platform that vibrates may improve circulation, flexibility, and potentially reduce pain.

Benefits of Sound and Vibration Techniques:

- Non-invasive and Drug-Free: These techniques offer a safe and natural approach to pain management and relaxation.
- Reduced Stress and Anxiety: Sound and vibration therapy can promote relaxation and reduce stress hormones, which can contribute to pain perception.
- Improved Sleep Quality: Relaxation techniques like listening to calming music can promote better sleep, aiding in overall recovery.
- Muscle Relaxation: Vibration therapy can help relax tense muscles, reducing discomfort and improving flexibility.

Things to Consider:

- Research is ongoing: While promising, the research on the effectiveness of sound and vibration therapy for pain management is still evolving.
- Individualized Effects: The effectiveness of these techniques can vary depending on the individual and the specific condition.
- Consulting a healthcare professional: If you're considering using sound or vibration therapy for pain management, consult your doctor or physical therapist to discuss if it's appropriate for your specific needs.

Subsection 9.4: Sound and Vibration Techniques

Overall, sound and vibration techniques offer a valuable and complementary approach to pain management and relaxation. By incorporating these techniques into your routine, you may experience reduced pain, improved sleep, and a more relaxed state of mind.

Subsection 9.5: Somatic Dance Movements and Somatic Yoga Integration

Somatic dance and somatic yoga, while having distinct approaches, share a common focus: cultivating body awareness and mindful movement. Integrating these practices can create a well-rounded experience that benefits your physical, mental, and emotional well-being.

Somatic Dance Movements:

- **Focus**: Explores movement through a lens of body sensations and internal experiences.
- **Emphasis**: Improvisation, playfulness, and expressing emotions through movement.
- **Benefits**: Increased body awareness, emotional release, and creative expression.

Somatic Yoga:

- **Focus**: Utilizes yoga postures (asanas) with a mindful exploration of internal sensations.
- **Emphasis**: Alignment, breathwork, and connecting movement with the breath.
- **Benefits**: Improved flexibility, mobility, reduced stress, and a deeper mind-body connection.

Integration:

Here's how you can combine somatic dance and somatic yoga for a holistic experience:

- Warm-up: Begin with somatic movement explorations. Move slowly, focusing on internal sensations like breath, muscle engagement, and joint movement.
- Somatic Yoga Flow: Transition into gentle yoga postures, emphasizing proper alignment and breathwork. Pay attention to how your body feels in each pose, rather than achieving perfect form.
- Somatic Dance Exploration: After holding yoga postures, return to free movement. Explore how the yoga poses have affected your body awareness and use that newfound awareness to guide your dance.
- Cool-down: End with gentle stretches and mindful breathing, integrating the sensations from both practices.

Subsection 9.5: Somatic Dance Movements and Somatic Yoga Integration

Benefits of Integration:

- Deeper Body Awareness: Combining the movement exploration of somatic dance with the mindful breathwork of somatic yoga can create a profound understanding of your body.
- Enhanced Emotional Expression: Somatic dance allows you to express emotions freely, while somatic yoga provides a safe space to process and release them.
- Improved Flexibility and Mobility: The combination can enhance your flexibility and range of motion, improving your overall physical well-being.
- Stress Reduction and Relaxation: Both practices promote relaxation and stress reduction, leading to a calmer and more centered state.

Getting Started:

Here are some tips for integrating somatic dance and somatic yoga:

- Find a Somatic Dance or Yoga Class: Look for classes specifically labeled as "somatic" or "movement exploration."
- Online Resources: There are many online resources offering guided somatic dance sessions and somatic yoga routines.
- Start Slowly: Begin with short sessions (10–15 minutes) and gradually increase the duration as you become more comfortable.
- Listen to Your Body: Focus on your internal sensations and adjust your movements accordingly. Don't push yourself beyond your limits.

Remember: The beauty of this integration lies in the journey itself. Embrace the exploration, prioritize body awareness, and enjoy the process of connecting with yourself through movement.

Subsection 9.6: Maintaining Spinal Health and Correct Posture

Maintaining spinal health and correct posture are crucial for overall well-being. Here's a breakdown of key strategies to keep your spine happy and your posture aligned:

Posture Power:

- Stand Tall: Imagine a string gently pulling the crown of your head upwards. Keep your shoulders relaxed and down, and avoid slouching.
- Neutral Spine: Maintain the natural curves of your spine. Avoid hunching your back or arching your lower back excessively.
- Screen Awareness: When using a computer, ensure your monitor is at eye level and your forearms are supported on a comfortable surface.

Strengthening Support:

- Core Powerhouse: Engage your core muscles throughout the day. Simple exercises like pelvic tilts and planks can strengthen your core, which stabilizes your spine.
- Targeted Exercises: Regularly perform exercises that target your back, chest, and abdominal muscles. These will help maintain proper posture and support your spine.

Subsection 9.6: Maintaining Spinal Health and Correct Posture

Ergonomic Enhancements:

- Supportive Seating: Invest in an ergonomic chair with good lumbar support and adjust it to fit your body properly.
- Standing Breaks: If you sit for extended periods, take frequent standing breaks to prevent stiffness and promote circulation in your back.

Movement Matters:

- Regular Exercise: Engage in activities that promote flexibility and mobility, such as yoga, Pilates, or swimming.
- Mindful Movement: Be mindful of your posture throughout the day, especially during activities like lifting objects or carrying a bag.

Lifestyle Habits:

- Maintain a Healthy Weight: Excess weight can put strain on your spine. Maintaining a healthy weight reduces stress on your spinal joints.
- Hydration is Key: Staying hydrated keeps your spinal discs healthy and functioning properly.

Sleeping for Spinal Support:

- Choose the Right Mattress: A supportive mattress that conforms to your body's curves is crucial. Opt for a medium-firm mattress that keeps your spine aligned.
- Sleeping Positions: Side sleeping with a pillow between your knees is generally considered a good position for spinal health. Avoid sleeping on your stomach, which can strain your neck and lower back.

Mind-Body Connection:

- Stress Management: Chronic stress can contribute to muscle tension and poor posture. Practice stress-reduction techniques like yoga, meditation, or deep breathing to keep your body relaxed.
- Body Awareness: Throughout the day, take a moment to check your posture. Notice any slouching or tension in your shoulders and adjust accordingly.

Supportive Gear:

- Lumbar Support Pillow: Using a lumbar support pillow while driving or sitting for long periods can help maintain the natural curve of your lower back.
- Adjustable Standing Desk: Consider using an adjustable standing desk to alternate between sitting and standing throughout the workday. This can help reduce strain on your spine and improve circulation.

Complementary Therapies:

- Massage Therapy: Regular massages can help release muscle tension and improve flexibility in your back and core.
- Alexander Technique: This mind–body technique focuses on improving posture by retraining your movement patterns.

Early Intervention:

- Don't Ignore Pain: If you experience persistent back pain, don't ignore it. Early diagnosis and treatment of any underlying conditions can help prevent future problems.
- Regular Checkups: Schedule regular checkups with your doctor or physiotherapist to monitor your spinal health and address any concerns early on.

Remember, maintaining good spinal health is an ongoing process. By incorporating these tips into your lifestyle and maintaining a proactive approach, you can prevent future problems and ensure a healthy, pain-free spine for years to come.